NUMBER 425

THE ENGLISH EXPERIENCE

ITS RECORD IN EARLY PRINTED BOOKS
PUBLISHED IN FACSIMILE

The publishers acknowledge their gratitude to the Curators of the Bodleian Library, Oxford for their permission to reproduce the Library's copy, Shelfmark: 8°R.16Art BS.

Library of Congress Catalog Card Number: 77-38145

S.T.C.No. 1199

Collation: A-C^8

Published in 1972 by

Theatrvm Orbis Terrarvm Ltd.,
O.Z.Voorburgwal 85, Amsterdam

&

Da Capo Press Inc.
-a subsidiary of Plenum Publishing Corporation-
277 West 17th Street, New York N.Y. 10011

Printed in the Netherlands

ISBN 90 221 0425 7

A
Short Diſcourſe of the three kindes of PEPPERS in common vſe, and certaine ſpecial medicines made of the ſame, tending to the preſeruation of health.

by W. Bailey.

1588

To the right worship[ful]
Sir John Cowper knight

AS in former yeeres at this season I haue been alwaies careful to shew my special affection towards yor w[orship] by offering som present, appertaining to the preseruatiõ of your health: so at this time, right w[orshipful] in token of a good and prosperous newe yeere, (God grant you many) I haue emboldened my selfe to exhibite vnto you in our vulgar toong, this short discourse of the three kindes of Peppers, and of three medicines cõpounded of the same, greatly commended by Galen in his books De sanitate tuenda; which being vsed in right order, with discretion, will vndoubtedly bring three waies commoditie to the continuance of your heath. For it is certaine that most men in this our countrey through our maner of feeding, do gather in *the ſtomacke and in the first veines many crude and vndigeſted humours, which do often occaſion lacke of appetite, groſſe windines, diſtentions in the ſides, and many waies greeuous paines; and ſometimes vnnaturall vomits: which crudities carried farther into the body, doo breede obſtructions, tympanies, feuers, and other dangerous diſeaſes. The due conſideration hereof, may eaſily inferre how neceſſary to health in this our region the vſe of pepper is, and what commodity may accrew by conuenient vſe of the three medicines made thereof. For firſt the medicine termed* diatrion pipereon, *by conſent of all writers, hath facultie to warme the ſtomacke, to dry ſuperfluous moiſture, to further concoction, to diſcuſſe winde, to ripen crude humours, and is cōmended aboue all other medicaments, that in performing of theſe actions it doth no way ouerheate the liuer, nor diſtemper the bloud. The ſecond medicine termed* diaſpoliticon, *keepeth the belly looſe, and doth carry by the ſtoole, crude, corrupt, and naughtie humours, cut groſſe and thicke phlegme, keepeth cleane the belly and guts. The third medicine termed* diacalaminthe, *hauing more ſubtiltie in ſubſtance doth penetrate farther, and ſo doth concoct and expell not onely the crudities of the belly and of the firſt veines, but alſo doth digeſt, extenuate, diſcuſſe, and by vrine carieth the excrements of the inner*

ner

ner veines, clenſeth the bloud, and keepeth clean the habite of the body by ſweate and perſpiration through the skin. That in very truth Galen had iuſt cauſe ſo greatly to commende theſe three medicines as moſt conuenient to preſerue health. For I do not reade in all our authors of a more conuenient meanes to continue health, than the apte and due vſe of theſe three medicines, which in propulſing of diſeaſes, and in reforming of the ſtate of the body, may be reſembled to the triumuiri in the common-wealth of Rome. Wherefore I remaine to the almightie a daily orator ſo to proſper the effects of theſe medicines, that the ſame commodities may come vnto [redacted]

yo[illegible] *which our authors do attribute vnto them, that your yeeres may be inlarged to extreame age.*

* * *

[illegible]

walter Bailey

Of the Spice called
Pepper.

THAT kind of ſpice which of the Greeke authors is called πέ-περι, the Latin writers do name *Piper*, and the apothecaries do terme the ſame as the Latiniſts. After the Arabike ſpeech in Auicen it is read *Fulful*, in Serapio *Fulfel.* Garcia a phyſician to the viceroy of India, doth write, that the Arabians in theſe daies do call it *Fulfil*: and he addeth, that the greateſt quantitie of this ſpice is nowe brought into Europe, out of the prouince of Malauar: and that the ſame is in that countrie language named *Molonga.* We in Engliſh do call it pepper: and much vſe of this ſpice with vs is, in making broths, and in conditing meates.

The kinds of Pepper.

HEer it is to be noted, that many herbs of our writers are termed by the name of pepper. For the herbe called in

Latin *Persicaria*, in Engliſh Culrage, is of ſome named water pepper. The ſeede alſo of the herbe called Chamelea, is knowen to the herbarians by the name of hil pepper. Likewiſe the herbe which we call Stonecrop, is alſo named mouſe pepper. And ſom do cal diptander, herbe pepper, and ſome ſauery pepperwort. So the latter writers ſhew many other herbs vnder the name of pepper, and vnder pepperwort. For they refer to pepper euery kind of herbe which doth bite the toong as pepper doth. And beſide the three kindes of pepper, which are beſt knowen by that name, we do read in the latter writers of ſome other kinds vnder that name : and ſo we read of pepper out of Æthiopia, which is of the learned rather referred to that ſpice which is called Carpeſium, than to any kind of pepper. But properly and in true ſpeech, this word in Latin *Piper*, and in Engliſh pepper, is to be vnderſtood of one of the three peppers in common vſe, of which one is named white pepper, the other blacke pepper, the third long pepper. Of the which three kinds, and not of the other things falſly named peppers, that confection ſo greatly commended in cold affections of the ſtomack, called *Dia-*

trion

trion pipereon, is made, and kept in our Apothecaries ſhops. So that theſe three kindes of peppers moſt properly do deſerue the name of pepper, and are ſo moſt conueniently called: and the other things are rather by ſimilitude ſo termed, for yeelding ſome taſte like pepper, and therfore neuer knowen by the name of pepper without ſome addition, as *Piper montanum*, *Piper murinum*, *&c.* So that when we do read in any author this word *Piper*, or in Engliſh pepper without addition, we muſt vnderſtand the ſame of one of theſe three peppers.

The nauigations in theſe latter yeeres made by the Portingales into the eaſt Indians, and by the Spaniards into the weſt Indians, hath made manifeſt to vs, how greatly the old authors, I meane Dioſcorides, Galen, Plinie, Auicenna, Serapio, and other writers of the former time were deceiued in and about the hiſtorie of pepper. For firſt, all the ancient writers in their monuments haue deliuered to vs, that the three kindes of pepper in common vſe are all three the fruit of one tree. For (ſay they) the pepper tree doth bear a long fruit, like vnto that which doth hang in haſell nut trees, and birch trees. And

they

they affirme, that this long fruit is the first rudiment of the pepper, which is called long pepper : after that this fruit being more ripe is disclosed, they take the seeds contained in it to be the white pepper, & the blacke pepper: such graines which are not perfectly ripe, they supposed to be white pepper, and those which are perfectly ripe, to be blacke pepper. So they concluded, that these three kinds were all the fruit of one tree, and differed only in that one was not so ripe as the other. But by the nauigations of the Portingals, and of the Spaniards into those countries, in which these pepper trees do growe, it is euident and well knowen, that the trees which do yeeld these three spices are diuers in kind. For the trauellers into those countries which haue seene the trees, and gathered the fruits, do witnes, that not one and the same tree, but diuers and different do beare these spices. And that the plants which do beare white pepper and blacke pepper are not trees of any bignes, but weake shrubs, which do clime vp by other trees, as an Iuie doth in this our countrie. And haue leaues like to the apple tree called *Malum Assyrium*, and do carrie their fruit in clusters, like the clu-

sters

ſters of grapes of vine trees, which are alway greene vntill they wax ripe. And Garcia, who liued in theſe parts, writeth, that the plant which yeeldeth the white pepper, doth in kind differ from that which beareth the blacke pepper, and yet are ſo like, that no man can know the one from the other, but they which do dwell there. For (ſaith he) they do ſo differ, as the vine tree which beareth the white grape, doth differ from that which yeeldeth the red grape: and as we cannot know the difference of theſe vine trees, but when the grape is ripe, ſo we cannot diſcerne the plant which yeeldeth the white pepper, from that which beareth the blacke pepper: and yet (ſaith he) it is certaine, that the ſame tree, which bringeth foorth the blacke pepper, doth not yeeld the white pepper. He ſaith alſo, that the white pepper tree is not ſo common in theſe countries as the other is, and that the ſame is not to be ſeene, but in certaine places of Malauar and Malachæ. The ſame Garcia writeth, that the tree, of which long pepper is gathered, doth greatly differ from the other forenamed pepper trees: and that long pepper is a fruit depending of the tree in like ſort, as we ſee things to

hang

hang downe in our hasell nut trees,and in our birch trees: and that this fruit wil neuer yeeld either white or blacke pepper. By this discourse we do vnderstand, that the pepper tree is not like to the Iuniper tree,as Plinie writeth in his 12.boke. And Garcia also saith, that the roote of the pepper tree is very little. So that it is not like to ginger, as some beleeued in Dioscorides time, nor like to the roote of Costus as Dioscorides writeth. And heerby also we are to vnderstand that the old saying is fabulous and vntrue, that pepper is made blacke with fire. For the marchants which brought the peppers, said,that serpents and venemous beasts did vse much to be vnder these pepper trees, and that they were driuen to fray away those serpents with making fires vnder the trees, before they durst gather the peppers, and so the pepper was made black by the fire. But now we learne by the histories penned by the latter writers, that all this is vntrue, and that blacke pepper is of that colour by his owne kinde,when it is ripe: and so that white pepper is of his owne kind, euen of that colour when it is ripe. As the red grape hath that colour naturally when it is ripe, and the white

grape

grape keepeth his colour euen to his full ripenes. Wherefore those writers were much deceiued, which affirmed, that white and black pepper were of one tree: and that white pepper was the fruit not throughly ripe, and that blacke pepper was the same perfectly ripe. For (say they) as in our country, when we gather apples, all of the same tree are not of like ripenes, some not full ripe, some full ripe, some ouer ripe, and all are gathered at one time: so, say these men, when the marchants do gather pepper, some graines are throughly ripe, and they black and wrinkled, some not full ripe, and they whiter in colour, and smoothe not wrinkled. But it appeereth by that which they haue deliuered to vs, which haue seene and gathered both these kinds of peppers, that they are gathered of seuerall trees, and that ech doth perfectly ripe in his kind, and ech retaine his colour: the white graine when it is ripe keepeth the white colour, and the blacke pepper when it is ripe keepeth his blacke colour: Euen as the white grape being ripe remaineth white, and the red grape red, and yet ech do come of seuerall vine trees different in kinde. So we are to thinke of these kinds of pepper, that ech

doth

doth come of his proper tree,and each ful ripe retaineth his naturall colour : the white pepper his, and the blacke his colour, as doth euidently appeere by that which Garcia hath written in his firſt booke *De aromat. Indiæ.*

That the Greeke & ancient writers did erre in expreſſing the hiſtory of theſe peppers,it is no maruel: for in that their coũtries were far diſtant from the prouinces frõ whence theſe peppers came, that they themſelues could not ſearch out a truth, but followed the report of marchants, which tell many vntruthes, they were eaſily deceiued, and ſo did ſet down in their bookes for verities many vntrue relations of the marchants.

But that the Arabians did commit the ſame errors, whoſe countrie was not far diſtant from the places where pepper doth grow,their groſſe negligence in ſearching the true knowledge of ſimples, can not be excuſed,who would rather followe heerein that which was written by the Grecians, than themſelues ſearch out a truth.

Matthiolus in his commentaries vpon Dioſcorides witneſſeth,that many pepper trees are ſet to be ſeene at Naples, and at at Venice, and diuers affirme, that theſe trees are planted in diuers places in Spain and in Portingall. But I could neuer vnderſtand that any pepper tree was at any time brought into England. I haue often ſeene at Poole in Dorſetſhire, and alſo in London,the whole cluſters of pepper preſerued in brine and in ſalt : theſe cluſters are long and thin, not ſo thicke togither as the cluſters of grapes.

Long pepper is to be ſeene in euery ſhop: for the whole fruit is brought by the marchants gathered togither like ſcales, rough & vneuen, biting the toung like the other peppers.

We do read of another kind of pepper brought out of the Indians, which the Portingals called *Piemento de Rabo*, in Latin *Piper caudatum*, and may be engliſhed taile pepper.Cluſius in his annotations in Garcia, ſeemeth to haue known this kind of pepper, and ſaith that it is like to the cubebs, and that it hangeth in cluſters, is very ſpicie,and hath a little ſtalke or ſtem. This kind is not now brought : for the king of Portingall did forbid any to bring it, fearing leaſt it might decay the price and ſale of the other kindes.

Monardis alſo in his booke *De plantis*

Indiæ,

India, maketh mention of another kind of long pepper, different from the common long pepper, and is much hotter than the common long pepper, and more pleaſant to the taſte than blacke pepper. Where the latter writers in the hiſtorie of pepper do diuide long pepper into the garden and wild, this kind written of by Monardis is ſuppoſed to be the wilde long pepper, and the common long pepper, the garden or domeſticall.

The latter writers in the hiſtorie of pepper, do write of another kind of pepper, which they call *Piper corniculatum*, ſome call it *Siliquaſtrum*, which may bee engliſhed, Codded pepper, bicauſe it beareth his graines in a cod or huske: and they deſcribe this kinde to haue leaues like to the herbe called Nightſhade, a ſquare ſtalk of colour greene, ful of ioints, white flowers, and after them commeth the cod, at the firſt greeniſh, and after red, with a perfect ſmoothnes and ſlikenes: within that cod are flat graines, whitiſh, yellow, more biting in taſte than pepper. Theſe cods are not alway of one forme: for in ſome of the plants they are greater and longer, in ſome leſſer and ſhorter: and the leſſer kind they call pepper of Braſilia: the

the greater they call pepper of Calecut, named after the countries from whence they are brought. The herbarians of our time do witnes, that this plant is ſet in diuers places in Italie, Spaine and Portingal: for that it is a goodly plant and faire to the eie, and the graines are vſed for pepper all the yere, and are thought to commend meates condited with them, better than common pepper. I did neuer ſee the plant, but the cods are common in the Apothecaries ſhops. It is ſuppoſed of many, that the olde Greeke authors haue not written any thing of this plant, but Actuarius ſeemeth to ſpeake of this kinde of pepper, vnder the name of *Capſicum*. Amatus in his commentaries vpō Dioſcorides affirmeth, that this kinde of pepper is that which Auicen in 2. tract. lib. 2. cap. 746. called *Zinziber caninum*. Thus much of the true hiſtorie of pepper, as well out of the old as latter writers.

How to chooſe pepper.

DIoſcorides writing of three kinds of pepper, doth giue ſignes and notes to chooſe onely blacke pepper : for that as it ſeemeth in his time deceit was onely vſed in that kind of pepper. For Dioſcorides writeth, that amongſt blacke pepper are found certaine ſeedes or graines light, and emptie, which he calleth *Breſma*, and Plinie ſaith they are termed *Brechmaſis*, which word doth ſound, ſeeds vttered before their time. For (ſaith he) by vnſeaſonable time the graines ſometimes do wither, and ſo are emptie, hauing in them no ſubſtance. But Garcia ſaith, that while he did dwel among the Indians, he inquired, & could not learne of any ſuch name, yet acknowledgeth, that ſuch graines like to pepper are often found amongſt pepper, and are not eaſily knowen from pepper, but that they are light, and broken do yeeld no ſubſtance as pepper doth. Wherfore as in Dioſcorides time, ſo rather in this our age, we ought to be diligent in the choiſe of pepper, and to haue ſome notes or ſignes to chooſe the good from the bad, and to know the beſt pepper. Dioſcorides commendeth pepper when the graines are heauie, full, whole, not much wrinkled, new, not full of duſt. And Galen in 4. *De ſanit. tuend.* adddeth, which hath not a very thinne, nor yet a groſſe and thicke skin.

Serapio praiſed white pepper, which hath

hath a white colour,and the latter writers ſay,the whiter the better,which is ſmooth and not wrinkled. Galen in 4.*De ſanit.tuend.*ſaith,that thoſe grains are beſt, which are fulleſt and greateſt.

Serapio alloweth of long pepper,which when it is broken,doth ſhew his ſubſtance compacted, and his graines thicke ioined togither, which do bite the toong with ſenſible heate.Galen in the ſaid booke *De ſanit.tuend.*addeth, that long pepper muſt be whole, and not haue any holes in it, and not ſophiſticated. For(ſaith he) the marchants do bring two ſorts counterfeited, the one is the bud of an herbe,the other is made in Alexandria by art. And in his booke *De theriaca ad Piſonem*,he telleth the maner of making of this counterfet long pepper. They forme it (ſaith he)of the length & bignes of this pepper, and then caſt to it the powder of the root of *Pyrethrum*, or of muſtard ſeed, & ſo deceiue the taſte. But theſe deceits are eaſily bewraied:for by taſte you may diſcern the right pepper from the buds of that herb, which are in form like to long pepper,but not in taſte:and ſo by taſting,you ſhal diſcern the one frő the other.For whoſoeuer wil with diligence obſerue the taſt of pepper, he ſhall eaſily iudge that pleaſant ſpicines which it yeeldeth with the biting. And Galen ſheweth how to diſcerne the counterfeited frõ the right, by putting it into water.For the counterfeited will diſſolue in water, and ſo the right and naturall will not diſſolue. Wherefore he concludeth, that if it hath the true taſte of pepper, and doth not diſſolue in water, nor hath holes in it, then that is good pepper. All writers do make this for a ſigne of good long pepper, when it hath no holes: for in deed this pepper is moiſter than any other kinde, and therefore will ſooner mould and waxe muſtie than the other, and ſo will quickly be woorme eaten,and full of holes.

Of the temperament of Pepper.

Dioſcorides and Galen do yeeld to all the kinds of pepper a faculty to heat and to drie, but neither of them do declare in what degree they do heate and drie. After that Auerrhois in *lib. Simplic.* had pronounced long pepper to be moiſter than the other: And that white pepper was not come to his ripenes, and that black pepper was full ripe:He concludeth both

both kinds to be hot in the third degree, and as ſome ſay in the fourth degree. Auicen in lib.2. tract.2. intreating of white and blacke pepper generally, affirmeth pepper to be hot and drie tending toward the fourth degree. And in the very next chapter handling of long pepper, he writeth that it is hot in the third degree, and drie in the ſecond. Dioſcorides doth not appoint the degrees of heat and drines to euery kind of pepper, yet handleth each very diſtinctly, ſaying, that long pepper doth more ſtrongly bite: and bicauſe it is taken from the tree before it is ripe, therfore it remaineth a little bitter. Blacke pepper, bicauſe it is perfectly ripe, therefore it is well ſauored, ſharper than white pepper,& ſo more pleaſing to the mouth, and more profitable to condite meates. The white pepper remaining a little bitter,is not ſo ſtrong as the blacke. By this Dioſcorides concludeth,that blacke pepper is the hotteſt, and beſt of all; next to it is long pepper, and that the weakeſt is the white pepper. Galen doth ſeeme heerin to diſſent from Dioſcorides. For Galen in 8.*ſimpl.med.facult.* doth put long pepper to be moiſter than the reſt, bicauſe it is the yoong fruit,and therefore doth ſoone waxe woorme eaten. And after affirmeth, that white pepper is more ſharpe and biting than the blacke, and giueth this reaſon of his aſſertion: for that blacke pepper is euer heated and dried with the ſun by long tarrieng vpon the tree: for heerby many of his hot and fierie parts do breath out, the rather bicauſe pepper is of a thin ſubſtance, that his hot parts will quickly conſume and breath out: and ſo he concludeth, that bicauſe white pepper is not ſo heated and dried by the ſun, but doth retaine and keepe al his hote parts, therefore it is the hotter, more biting, and the beſt pepper, contrarie to Dioſcorides aſſertion. Braſſauolus Muſa going about to reconcile this controuerſie in Galen, by diſtinguiſhing of the Greeke word δριμυτέρον. For in that white pepper hath plentie of moiſture in it, therefore it biteth ſtronger, and leaueth the ſharpe and biting qualitie to continue longer: and in that reſpect it may be ſaid to be hotter than the blacke pepper, hauing little moiſture, and that much extenuated by the heate of the ſunne, doth bite quicklier, deeper, and ſharper: but bicauſe the heate of his biting doth not ſo long continue, therefore it ſeemeth not ſo hot as the blacke,

and

and yet for that it biteth deeper, therfore Dioſcorides writeth, that it is hotter and ſtronger than the blacke. And if to trie the truth heereof, a man will taſte both kinds of pepper, ſurely he ſhall manifeſtly perceiue the difference of them both. And ſo in the one ſenſe white pepper may be ſaid to be hotter and more biting, as Galen writeth: and in the other ſenſe blacke pepper may be thought to exceede the white as Dioſcorides affirmeth. But where Dioſcorides ſaith, that white pepper is weaker than long pepper and black pepper, bicauſe it not being ful ripe is acerbious or more tart: ſurely his argument is not perfect. For as he putteth white pepper not ſo ripe as blacke, ſo he maketh long pepper not ſo ripe as white pepper. And ſo it muſt follow after his opinion, that long pepper ſhould be weaker than white, and white than blacke pepper. So Hippocrates is deceiued in his owne reaſoning. But in that it is now certaine, that theſe kinds do not differ, that the one is riper than the other, but each is ripe and perfect in his kinde: theſe arguments of more or leſſe ripenes, do take no place, and are of no efficacie: bicauſe that by taſte it is euident, that white pepper doth bite the toong more, and the biting doth continue longer: therefore we may iustly ſay that white pepper is the hotter. And for that Galen lib.9. *De compoſit.ſec.loc.* in the medicine of Philo affirmeth, that white pepper is better for the ſtomacke than blacke pepper. And in 4.*De ſanit.tuend.*he ſaith,that white pepper doth ſtrēgthen the ſtomack aboue the other kinds. Surely the Friers writing vpon Meſue do truly counſell Apothecaries when pepper ſimply is read,to take white pepper.

Notwithſtanding in ſome affects long pepper is to be preferred before the other kinds, as Galen witneſſeth lib.4. *De ſanit. tuend.* where he counſelleth to giue long pepper to them which haue their ſides blowen vp with wind, and which do turne all they eate to wind. For (ſaith he) long pepper doth diſſolue the groſnes of wind, & caſteth downe by the belly ſuch matter which doth ſtay in the ſides.

By this diſcourſe it appeereth,that the Arabians did truly ſet white and blacke pepper in the vttermoſt point of the third degree of heate and drines, or in the beginning of the fourth degree. And Galen confirmeth the ſame when he doth write, that white and blacke pepper do ſtrongly

heate

heate and drie.

And with good reaſons the ſame Arabikes do ſet long pepper in the third degree of heate, and not beyond the ſecond degree of drying. For in that by all writers conſent this kind is moiſter than the other, therefore it cannot drie ſo much as the other: for the drying qualitie muſt needs be ſomwhat obtunded by the moiſture which is in this kind. And therefore long pepper taſted doth not by and by bite ſtrongly, but after it is a little chewed, and then the biting doth laſt longer. And we may heerby alſo gather, that long pepper is not ſo ſubtill of ſubſtance as the other kinds are.

Garcia writeth, that Emperikes amongſt the Arabians & Perſians do hold opinion, that pepper is cold: which opinion doth alſo preuaile amongſt the common ſort in this our countrie. For it is a common ſaying, that pepper is hot in the mouth, but cold in operation. But for as much as we do trie the qualitie of medicines by taſte, theſe men do ſhew their ignorance, in calling that cold in operation, which is hot in the mouth.

The

The temperament of Siliquaſtrum, or Indian Pepper.

THe Indian pepper called alſo Siliquaſtrum, is accounted hot and drie in the fourth degree, and therefore doth very effectually breake wind, doth heat and ſtrengthen the inward parts, and is verie good for the breaſt.

The vertues and faculties of Pepper.

DIoſcorides, Plinie, Auicenna, and Serapio do recite and number manie vertues and medicinal properties of theſe kindes of peppers, which I leaue the reader to peruſe in their books. The cheefeſt vſe of peppers is in cold affects of the ſtomacke, and of other parts which do ſerue for nutrition. For euery kind of pepper doth greatly helpe concoction, diſcuſſe wind, and doth occaſion all groſſe and ſlimie humors to diſcend ſooner. And to this purpoſe many medicines deuiſed by phyſicians of theſe kinds of peppers are kept in Apothecaries ſhops, but amongſt other Galen in his 4. booke *De ſanit. tuend.*

doth

doth chiefly cõmend three ſorts. And the medicine termed *Diatrion pipereon*, in that it is confected of the three kindes of pepper, beareth the bell, and is reputed in the firſt place. And then he commendeth the medicine called *Diacalaminthe* : & thirdly, that which is vſed vnder the name of *Diaſpoliticon* : notwithſtanding each of theſe medicines is not good to the ſelfeſame affects, neither are they in like ſort & times to be vſed. Touching *Diatrion pipereon*, it is famous for to help concoction, to diſcuſſe wind, and to do good againſt cold affects of the ſtomacke, and yet not to heate the liuer or the blood, wherin conſiſteth a ſingular propertie of this medicine. For it is agreed vpõ by all authors, that the heat of this medicine is extinguiſhed in the belly, and the firſt veines, & is not carried into the whole bodie, as the heat of the medicine called *Diacalaminthe* is; ſo termed, for that it receiueth the herbe called Calaminth, as Gal. writeth in the ſaid booke *De ſanit. tuend. cap.* 10. where he affirmeth, that *Diatrion pipereon* is to be giuen when crude and ſlimy humors are in the ſtomack and firſt veines, yea both before and after meate. The vſe of *Diacalaminthe* is, when we meane to warme further into the bodie,

bodie, and haue an intent to cut & make thin grosse humors in the veines. For *Diacalaminthe* doth thinne grosse and slimie things, breatheth out by the skin, prouoketh vrine, and the monethly sicknes in women. Therefore neither this medicine, neither *Diaspoliticon* ought to be vsed after meate, bicause they two hasten distribution, and so do hinder concoction: whereby we may conclude, that the medicine *Diatrion pipereon* may with most safetie be vsed after meate to helpe concoction. And to this intent Galen doth counsell to haue in a readines this medicine prepared in two maner of waies: the one simple, as cōsisting of fewest things; the other more compound: the simplier is soonest concocted; the other by reason of the number of simples is harder to be digested. And therefore the simplier is best for them which do not well concoct their meate, and do finde some cold temperament in the stomacke and bellie, and so do gather much slimie flegme: and the other by reason of many simples in it, is harder to be altered of nature, and so doth remaine longer in the stomacke when it is taken. So Galen doth best cōmend the frequent vse of *Diatrion piperēō* to remoue crudities

in

in the ſtomacke and firſt veines. The other which is more compound, hath his beſt vſe in fluxes from the head to the breaſt. In theſe our daies the medicine *Diatrion pipereon* is in vſe, made in both waies. In compounding the ſimplier, our Apothecaries do follow Nicolaus Myrepſicus, & ſo do make the medicine in maner as followeth: Taking of each of the three peppers one ounce, of

ginger,
thyme,
aniſe ſeedes,
perſley ſeedes } of each halfe an ounce.

This deſcription commeth nigh to the *Diatrion pipereon* of Galen. For there is no difference, but that Galen taketh of each kind of pepper fiftie drachmes, of ginger, thyme, aniſe ſeedes eight drachmes. Galen hath in his receit no perſley at all: yet Galen admoniſheth, that to 50. drachmes of each pepper, 16. drachmes of the other things may be added. And Galen willeth this medicine to be made with honie of Athens: in this our time it is compounded with ſugar. The other *Diatrion pipereon* more compound and medicinall is at this time made according to the deſcription of Meſue, in maner as followeth.

Take

Take of the three kinds of
pepper ʒ.6. ℈.ij.

ginger, anise ſeedes, thyme	ana. ʒ.ij. ℈.ij.
ſpikenard, amomum	ana. ʒ.j. ℈.j.
caſſia lignea, aſarum, enula camp. dried, perſley ſeeds ſeſeli	ana. ℈.ij.

ſaccharum albiſſimum q. ſ.

This is the ſame laborious confection ſet downe by Meſue, of which Galen maketh mention, lib.4.cap.11. *De ſanit.tuend.* For Galen in that place doth recite by name euery ſimple: ſaue that Galen in ſtead of Amomum, mentioneth the ſeeds of ammios. And where our authors do differ in opinion, what is the right Amomum, and all writers do agree, that we haue the right ammi: I adiudge it better in theſe daies to put in this receit the ſeeds of ammi, according as Galen preſcribeth, than amomum, as Meſue counſelleth. So you haue both medicines in vſe in our time made of three peppers, and

are

are to be ſold in the Apothecaries ſhops, vnder the name of *Diatrion pipereon*.

Diaſpoliticon.

THE medicine called *Diaſpoliticon* is moſt commended to looſe the belly: this medicine is compoſed of cummine ſeedes, pepper, rue, and that kinde of ſalt called *Salnitre*. And Galen aduiſeth to haue this medicine alſo prepared in two ſorts. Firſt to make it of the foreſaid ſimples mixed in equall parts, and ſo by reaſon of that ſalt, it wil looſe the belly more: the ſecond way to put to equall parts of the other things, but onely halfe the proportion of that kinde of ſalt. So will the medicine remaine longer in the ſtomack, and better further concoction, more digeſt crude and rawe humors, and wil leſſe make the bellie laxatiue.

Diacalaminthe.

GAlen in his fourth booke *De ſanitate tuend*. ca. 14. doth ſet downe the compoſition of the medicine called *Diacalaminthe*, in maner following.

Take

Take of calaminth,
of organy, or organmint, called Pulegiũ,
of persley, which groweth in stonie places, called Petroselinum,
of the herbe called Seseli,
of ech ℥.ij.

of persley seedes,
of the tops of thyme,
of ech ℥.iiij

of louage, ℥. 16.
of pepper, ℥. 48.

And Galen doth name the countries from which he counselleth to procure the simples, but in that they are not in these daies brought from those places, therefore it shall suffice to make choise of the best simples of this our countrie in confecting of this medicine : for this our countrie yeeldeth verie good of euerie sort.

In dispensing of this medicine, our Apothecaries do not follow this description of Galen, but their Apothecary booke confected by Nicolaus ; which composition doth differ from that of Galen in the doses of the simples, and that this of Nicolaus hath some mo simples than that of Galen.

Galen. The receite after Nicolaus is as followeth.

Take of calamints, organie, ſeſelios, blacke pepper, petroſelini	of ech ʒ.iij. ℈.ij.
leuiſtici.	ʒ.ij. ℈.j.
perſley ſeede	℈. j.
ammy ſeede, thime, anniſe ſeede, cinnamon, ginger.	of ech ℈.ij.

In this compoſition, perſley ſeeds, ammy, anniſe ſeedes, ginger, are mo then are ſet in the deſcription of Galen. Some learned men of our time do commend this receit of Nicolaus before that of Galen, bicauſe it hath mo ſimples : but for my part, I do rather allow of that receit of Galen, which for the paucitie of ſimples, is with leſſe labor concocted of them, which do take it, and to the intent of the medicine, it receiueth a ſufficient number of ſimples, ſo that they which are inſerted by Nicolaus ſeeme ſuperfluous.

Galen appointeth a proportion of the beſt and choſen honie, therewith to compounde this and the other medicines, which he willeth to be ſcummed with great diligence: and if the quantity of hony be increaſed, the medicine ſaith he will be more pleaſing. And he here ſetteth a rule which the apothecaries are to follow in compounding of medicines, to make them ſo pleaſant to the taſte as they can, without weakning of their ſtrength, or diminiſhing of their vertues. In theſe daies the moſt part of medicines are made vp with ſugar in ſteade of honie, for ſugar is more gratefull to the taſte, and many can not well away with honie. And honie is ſooner conuerted vnto choler than ſugar.

Touching the maner of making theſe medicines, Galen doth admoniſh, that they are not to be compounded in one and like ſort, for in ſome reſpects the ſimples are to be pounded finely, and ſerſed with a fine ſerſer. For ſaith he when things are finely beaten, they paſſe quickly into the whole body, things groſely powdered do ſtay longer in the belly, for the ſame cannot ſo eaſily paſſe through the little veines and ſmall pores of the body. In which reſpect things groſely powdered do more looſe the belly: when they are brought

brought into fine powder,they go ſooner into the body , and prouoke ſweate, and better mooue vrine,but do leſſe mooue to ſtoole. Therefore in compounding of the medicines called *Diacalaminthe* Galens counſell is to bring all the ſimples into fine powder,that the ſame may the better paſſe into all parts of the body,for the vſe of this medicine is, when we haue an intent to concoct and digeſt the crude and rawe humours in the inner veines and habite of the bodie,and ſo to euapore them by the pores of the skin, when we meane to prouoke ſweate, vrine, and the courſes of women,And therefore he will not haue this medicine often vſed after meate. In the medicine called *Diaſpoliticō*,al the ſimples muſt be pounded in groſſe maner,for ſo the medicine will more looſe the belly, and by ſtaieng longer in the ſtomack,further concoction , if the things be finely powdered into duſt : as the medicine will little or not at all make the belly laxatiue, ſo it will prouoke vrine and ſweate, to the intention of this medicine.

The like manner is to be obſerued in confecting of *Diatrion pipereon* , that if an intent be to haue the medicine ſtay in the ſtomacke and guts to warme thoſe parts, to digeſt crude humours in them, or to looſe the belly, the ſimples muſt be pounded groſſely: but if we haue a purpoſe to open obſtructions, to warme the inner veines, to prouoke vrine or ſweate: al-things muſt be beaten into fine powder. By which diſcourſe that queſtion is eaſily anſwered, which ſome latter writers do moue about the beating of the kindes of pepper, whether the ſame ought to be beaten finely or groſly. For ſome do affirme that pepper is alwaies to be beaten groſly, for ſo it will remaine longer time in the ſtomacke, and will the leſſe heate the liuer and the blood. Some other doo maintaine a contrary opinion, and that by Galen himſelfe, who in the 5. booke *De ſanit. tuend. cap.* 8. After meats which do bread ſtoppages in the body, take (ſaith he) the medicine called *Diacalaminthe*, and if you haue not it ready, take *Diatrion pipereon*: and if that be not at hand, take white pepper beaten into fine powder, & diligently ſerſed, & mingle the ſame with the meate, and ſprinkle it to your drinke. And in the ſame booke the 10. cap. Galen preſcribeth a ptiſane in which the duſt or fine powder of white pepper is mingled. And in the 6. booke *De ſanit. tuend. cap.* 14.

Galen

Galen giueth pepper alone, as finely powdered as may be. By these counsels of Galen, these men do conclude that pepper ought alway to be beaten into fine powder by Galens doctrine. Neuerthelesse, these men in mine opinion, do not with diligent care cōsider Galens intention in these and the like places, neither well haue marked the scope and cause why Galen in these places doth aduise to pound pepper into fine powder: for if they had well considered that Galen writeth : they might haue vnderstood, that he giueth pepper so finely beaten, to remoue the obstructions and stoppages, for so before he did admonish, that things beaten into thin powder passe into the body better, and sooner do remoue obstructions : and contrariwise, that which is grosly beaten, doth stay in the belly longer, and better warme those parts, better digest crude and rawe humors gathered in them, and do more effectually discusse wind: to these latter intents pepper is to be beaten grosly, especially in this our country, in which men commonly do feed vpon grosse and slimy meats, and so do heape in the parts of the belly and first veines, manie crude and grosse humors, that pepper ought in this region to be beaten moſt groſly, that it may therby be occaſioned to ſtay the longer in the belly, ſo to warme the ſame the better, and the better to concoct and extenuate ſuch groſſe and crude humors, for the heat of this medicine (as Galen writeth) is founded in ſo ſubtil a ſubſtãce, that the ſame is extinguiſhed before it can come to the liuer: then if you ſhall beate the medicine finely, the heate wil ſo ſoone be exhauſted and ſpent, that it will neither ſufficiently warme the belly, neither in good ſort concoct thoſe crude and rawe humors. Wherefore I do thinke it verie needfull for our apothecaries to pownd pepper alway groſly in the medicine *Diatrion pipereon*. For if we ſhall need withall to open obſtructions, we may preſcribe the medicine called *Diacalaminthe*, and ſo we may mingle it to *Diatrion pipereon*, or as occaſion ſerueth giue it alone: wherefore I hold it beſt to follow Galen his precept, which is, that alway things be powdered finely and in ſubtill manner when our purpoſe is to remoue obſtructions, or to digeſt, cut, and abſterge crude, rawe, ſlimy, and groſſe humors, which are in the inner veines and habite of the body, or meane to prouoke ſweat or vrine; but if

our

our meaning be to increaſe heate in the parts of the belly, to concoct humors there, and in the firſt veines, or to make the bellie looſe, then things are to be beaten in groſſe powder.

The priuate properties of the medicine called Diaſpoliticon.

THis medicine doth make the bellie looſe, and bringeth out meate, which corrupteth in the ſtomacke, and is ſpeciall good for them which haue a cold bellie, or declining to cold. For it maketh thinne groſſe phlegme, and expelleth flatulent winde. See Galen in the fourth booke *De ſanitate tuenda.*

The particular faculties and properties of Diatrion Pipereon.

D*Iatrion pipereon* is of great efficacie and doth much good in all colde diſeaſes of the ſtomacke, in ſower belkes, in quartaine feauers, in palſies, in euill affected liuers, in them which haue their bellies blowen vp with winde.

Diatrion pipereon confected after the deſcription of Meſues, is chiefly commended in fluxes, from the head to the breaſt, good generally to the coldnes of the cheſte, and to coughes, which do proceed of a colde cauſe.

That the excellent and rare vertues of this medicine called *Diatrion pipereon*, might the better be known, I thought good in this place to remember the reader what is written in the booke intituled *Secretorum*, which booke is aſcribed to Galen, in which booke we reade in this maner.

A certaine friend of mine being about the age of 70. yeeres, complained of a coldnes in all the parts of the bodie, inſomuch that his memorie failed him, and he had paine in his ioints, and then I made for him this medicine called *Diatrion pipereon*, and it was a wonder to ſee how he recouered in the ſpace of a fortnight. And I made triall in many which were ſicke of diſeaſes of the bladder, of the heade, and of the iointes, occaſioned by colde and crude humors: and it is found ſpeciall good in a cough of cold phlegme, in weakenes of the ſtomacke. For it breaketh groſſe winde, digeſteth meat, prouo-

keth

keth appetite , resolueth crude humours, strengtheneth the stomacke euerie way, restoreth memory,cleareth the voice,putteth backe grey heares , remedieth the goute which commeth of a colde cause : And in generall whosoeuer aged doth vse much this medicine,he shall not need any other helpe to preserue his health.

The priuate properties of the medicine called Diacalaminthe.

IT cutteth grosse and slimy humors,and occasioneth the same to be clensed by the skin by sweate,prouoketh vrine, and the monthly courses in women, as Galen witnesseth in the 4. booke *De sanit. tuend.* it is good for them which do abhor meat, for the vse of it prouoketh appetite, it remedieth the shortnes of breath, and helpeth them which finde a coldnes in their stomacks, and which haue their sides and bellies blowen vp with winde, as Mesue writeth.

The maner and particular vse of the foresaid medicines.

WHen many crude and rawe humors do abounde in the bellie

and

and firſt veines, that in that reſpect it will not be ſafetie to giue a purgatiue medicine, then is the cheefeſt vſe of *Diaſpoliticon*, for it then giuen will ſafely ſtir nature to expell thoſe humors by the ſiege. So in other caſes when ſo euer the belly is drie, and doth not hir dutie, then it is expedient to giue *Diaſpoliticon.*

The vſe of Diatrion pipercon, and of Diacalaminthe: out of Galen. 4. *De ſanit. tuend.*

WHen many raw and vndigeſted humors are gathered in and about the firſt veines, the ſame are to be cut and digeſted, and in ſo dooing ſpeciall care is to be had leſt the ſame be carried farther into the bodie. In this caſe *Diatrion pipereon* ſimple, is with moſt ſecuritie giuen. And it is not enough to giue it once or twiſe euery day, but it muſt be taken often, in the morning before meate, & after meat, & when they go to bed, a ſpoonfull at a time, and ſo to yonger folke and which haue leſſe need, the leſſer quantity: to elder and to them which haue more need, the bigger quantity, ſo to the mean,

the

the meaner quantitie is to be proportioned.

When crude humors are heaped in the inner veines,and in the habit of the body, the ſame are to be concocted, and alſo to be expelled by breathing the ſame thorough the pores of the skin, and to theſe intents there is not a more conuenient medicine knowen than *Diacalaminthe,* for it hath propertie to extenuate thicke,and ſlimy things, and then mooueth the ſame to be expelled by breathing out at the skin, and by vrine. And this medicine is not vnpleaſant to be taken, if a good proportion of honie be boiled with it, but where ſome do not like of ſweet things, and do abhor honie,to ſuch you muſt put the leſſe honie,yet oftentimes euen in this caſe it is good to boile good ſtore of honie,ſo you boile it well,for then the medicine will not be ouerſweet, and the honie well boiled doth leſſe offend the ſtomack. And the vſe of this medicine is in the morning after frictiō,before exerciſe,& before bathing. And you may vſe this medicine dry in powder without honie in ſteede of ſalt for ſauce to your meate, and you may put of it in a Ptiſane in ſteede of pepper.

This medicine is vſed not onely dry in ſteede

ſteede of ſalt, but alſo when honie is mixed, for euen ſo it may be vſed with meate, and ſo is it pleaſing to the taſte. But neither this, neither any other medicine which hath ſtrong facultie to further diſtribution, is to be taken after meate. For at that time nature goeth about concoction of meate taken, and not to diſtribute the ſame, therefore immediately after meate, endeuor muſt be to further concoctiō by giuing *Driatrion pipereon* ſimple, or to put ſome pepper powdered into your drinke.

If ſuch crudities hap to be not onely in the belly and firſt veines, but alſo in all other veines, yea in the fleſhie parts of the bodie: in this caſe at the beginning of the cure, it is beſt to vſe *Diatrion pipereon*, adding ſo much of the ſeeds of perſley growing in a drie & ſtonie ground, as is put of aniſe ſeedes, thyme, and ginger, and after the firſt day, or rather after the ſeconde day, you may put a little of *Diacalaminth*, and then in a while after mingle both, I meane *Diatrion pipereon*, and *Diacalaminth*, in equall parts, and in proceſſe of time increaſe the *Diacalaminthe*, ſo at the latter end of the cure, you may vſe *Diacalaminth* alone. So it is to be concluded in this, as in all maner of diets, when the effects are equall, the medicines to cure, are equally to be mixed, yet so that at the first greatest care be had of the crudities in the first veines, and at the latter end, of those crudities, which are in the other veines and habit of the bodie, in the middle time both are equally according to the effect to be mingled. Thus far Galen in his 4. booke *De sanitate tuenda.*

FINIS.